FAT LOSS EXTREME FOR SENIORS

Senior's Guide to Weight Reduction and Activation of
Metabolism for Healthy Lifestyle with Easy Exercise and
Delicious Recipes and Meal Plan.

Vince Cruise Sant

ABOUT THE BOOK

"Unlocking Your Best Self: A Lifelong Path to Health and Wellness" This book equips you with the tools you need to succeed as you age, from setting realistic objectives to controlling arthritis. Discover the secrets of mindful living, embrace technology for long-term transformation, and celebrate your journey to long-term happiness."

ABOUT THE AUTHOR

Introducing Vince Cruise Sant, a seasoned nutritionist with over a decade of dedicated experience in transforming lives through the power of balanced nutrition. With an extensive background in the field, Vince has emerged as a respected figure, dedicated to guiding individuals toward achieving their health and wellness aspirations.

With a wealth of practical knowledge and a deep understanding of nutrition and metabolism, Vince's expertise extends beyond theory. Having positively impacted the lives of more than 300 individuals, he stands as a testament to the tangible results his guidance brings.

Vince's approach transcends the conventional, recognizing the individuality of each person's journey toward well-being. His methodology seamlessly blends scientific insights with real-world application, ensuring that his advice is not only attainable but also sustainable.

Recognized as a trusted advisor and advocate for balanced nutrition, Vince Cruise Sant's commitment to empowering individuals is unwavering. His reputation as a compassionate and knowledgeable guide underscores his dedication to helping others unlock their full potential.

Whether you're a newcomer to the path of wellness or seeking to refine your existing practices, Vince's expertise will inspire and educate. Prepare to embark on a transformative journey led by a visionary who firmly believes that vibrant health is an achievable reality. With Vince's guidance, your pursuit of lasting well-being is poised for exceptional success.

TABLE OF CONTENTS

Maintaining Weight Loss and a Healthy LifestylE 66

INTRODUCTION

Why Fat Loss Matters for Seniors

As we age, maintaining a healthy weight becomes increasingly crucial for overall well-being and quality of life. Fat loss, when approached in a balanced and healthy manner, plays a pivotal role in ensuring seniors enjoy their golden years to the fullest. Let's delve into the reasons why fat loss matters for seniors:

1. Healthier Aging: Shedding excess body fat contributes to healthier aging. It reduces the risk of chronic diseases like heart disease, type 2 diabetes, and certain types of cancer, which become more prevalent in later life. A leaner body can help seniors manage these conditions more effectively.

2. Mobility and Independence: Carrying excess weight can strain joints and muscles, making it difficult to move comfortably. Weight loss can improve mobility, making everyday tasks, such as walking and climbing stairs, easier. This increased mobility fosters independence, a vital aspect of maintaining a high quality of life.

3. Enhanced Energy Levels: Fat loss can boost energy levels. Seniors who are at a healthy weight often find they have more vitality and enthusiasm for daily activities, from enjoying hobbies to spending quality time with loved ones.

4. Improved Heart Health: Losing fat can significantly reduce the risk of heart disease, a leading cause of death among seniors. Fat loss can lead to lower blood pressure and cholesterol levels, decreasing the strain on the heart and promoting cardiovascular health.

5. Enhanced Mental Well-being: Physical health and mental well-being are intertwined. Seniors who engage in weight loss activities often report improved mood, reduced symptoms of depression, and enhanced cognitive function. This positive mental state can lead to a more fulfilling life.

6. Better Sleep: Achieving and maintaining a healthy weight can alleviate sleep apnea and improve sleep quality. Adequate, restorative sleep is essential for seniors' physical and mental health.

7. Reduced Risk of Falls: Carrying excess weight increases the risk of falls and fractures, which can be particularly dangerous for seniors. Fat loss, coupled with strength training, can enhance balance and stability, reducing the likelihood of accidents.

8. *Less Stress on Organs:* Excess body fat places stress on vital organs like the liver and kidneys. Weight loss can reduce this burden, promoting better organ function and overall health.

9. *Medication Management:* Achieving a healthy weight can often reduce the need for medications or help seniors manage them more effectively. This can lead to fewer side effects and a higher quality of life.

10. *Increased Longevity:* Research suggests that maintaining a healthy weight can contribute to a longer life. Seniors who prioritize fat loss tend to experience fewer health issues and enjoy a more extended period of vitality.

Setting Realistic Goals

Setting realistic goals is a critical step in achieving success in any endeavor, including fat loss for seniors. Unrealistic goals can lead to frustration and demotivation, while realistic goals provide a clear path to success. Here's how to set realistic goals:

1. *Assess Your Current Situation:* Begin by taking an honest look at where you are right now. Consider factors like your current weight, fitness level, dietary habits, and any physical limitations you may have due to age or health issues.

2. *Understand Your Motivation:* Determine why you want to lose weight and get fit. Your motivation could be to improve your health, increase mobility, have more energy, or simply feel better about yourself. Understanding your "why" will help you set meaningful goals.

3. *Be Specific:* Set specific goals that are clear and well-defined. Instead of a vague goal like "I want to lose weight," say, "I want to lose 10 pounds in the next three months."

4. *Make goals measurable:* Your goals should be measurable so that you can track your progress. For example, "I will reduce my waist circumference by 2 inches" is measurable, whereas "I want a smaller waist" is not.

5. *Set attainable goals: While it's essential to challenge* yourself, your goals should be attainable. Consider your age, current fitness level, and any physical limitations. Setting unattainable goals can lead to frustration and disappointment.

6. *Set a Time Frame:* Determine a realistic time frame for achieving your goals. This adds a sense of urgency and helps you stay on track. For example, "I will lose 10 pounds in three months."

7. *Break It Down:* Divide your long-term goal into smaller, manageable milestones. This makes the process less overwhelming and allows you to celebrate small victories along the way.

8. *Consider Lifestyle Changes:* Understand that fat loss often requires lifestyle changes. Setting goals related to diet, exercise, and daily habits can help you stay on course.

9. *Stay Flexible:* Be willing to adjust your goals as needed. Life can be unpredictable, and circumstances may change. It's okay to modify your goals to suit your evolving needs and abilities.

10. *Track Your Progress:* Regularly monitor your progress using methods like tracking your weight, body measurements, or fitness achievements. Tracking keeps you accountable and motivated.

11. *Celebrate Achievements:* Celebrate your successes, no matter how small. Recognizing your progress boosts motivation and reinforces the belief that you can achieve your goals.

12. *Learn from setbacks:* Setbacks are a natural part of any journey. Instead of getting discouraged, view them as opportunities to learn and adjust your approach.

13. *Stay Positive:* Maintain a positive mindset throughout your journey. Self-compassion and a can-do attitude are essential for reaching your goals.

14. *Stay Consistent:* Consistency is key to achieving any goal. Stick to your plan, even on days when motivation is low. Consistent effort over time yields the best results.

CHAPTER 1

UNDERSTANDING SENIOR FAT LOSS

Age-Related Changes in Metabolism

As individuals age, several changes occur in their metabolism, which can impact their ability to manage weight effectively.

1. Slower Basal Metabolic Rate (BMR): BMR is the number of calories your body needs at rest to maintain basic functions like breathing and digestion. With age, BMR tends to decrease. This means that seniors may burn fewer calories at rest than they did when they were younger.

2. Loss of Muscle Mass: Muscle tissue is more metabolically active than fat tissue, meaning it burns more calories even when you're not exercising. Unfortunately, aging often leads to a gradual loss of muscle mass, which can contribute to a slower metabolism.

3. Reduced Physical Activity: Many seniors become less active as they age, which can further slowdown their metabolism. A sedentary lifestyle can result in muscle atrophy and decreased calorie expenditure.

4. *Changes in Hormones:* Hormonal fluctuations, particularly in menopause for women and declining testosterone levels for men, can influence metabolism. These changes can lead to an increase in body fat and a decrease in muscle mass.

The Importance of Lean Muscle Mass

Maintaining and even building lean muscle mass is crucial for seniors for several reasons:

1. *Increased Metabolism:* Muscle tissue burns more calories than fat tissue, even at rest. Having more muscle mass can help offset the natural decline in metabolism that occurs with age.

2. *Enhanced Mobility and Independence:* Strong muscles support better mobility, balance, and independence. This is essential for maintaining a high quality of life as you age.

3. *Better Blood Sugar Control:* Muscles play a role in regulating blood sugar levels. Having more muscle can help improve insulin sensitivity and reduce the risk of type 2 diabetes.

4. Bone Health: Resistance training, which builds muscle, also benefits bone health. This is particularly important for seniors who are at risk of osteoporosis.

5. Injury Prevention: Strong muscles can protect against injuries and falls, reducing the risk of fractures and other accidents common in seniors.

Hormonal Changes and Weight Gain

Hormonal shifts are a natural part of aging and can contribute to weight gain.

1. Menopause (in women): Menopause typically occurs in the late 40s or early 50s and is associated with a decrease in estrogen levels. This hormonal change can lead to increased fat storage, particularly around the abdomen.

2. Testosterone Decline (in Men): Testosterone levels tend to decline with age in men. This can result in reduced muscle mass, increased body fat, and a slower metabolism.

3. Stress Hormones: Chronic stress can elevate cortisol levels, a stress hormone that can promote fat storage, especially around the midsection.

4. *Thyroid Function:* Thyroid hormones play a role in metabolism. Some seniors may experience thyroid imbalances, which can affect weight regulation.

In summary, understanding the factors contributing to senior fat loss or gain is crucial for tailoring effective strategies. Seniors can combat age-related changes in metabolism by staying physically active, focusing on building and maintaining lean muscle mass, and adopting a well-balanced diet. Additionally, addressing hormonal changes through healthy lifestyle choices can help mitigate the risk of weight gain and associated health issues.

CHAPTER 2

NUTRITION FOR SENIORS

Balanced Eating for Weight Loss

Balanced eating forms the cornerstone of a successful and sustainable weight loss journey, particularly for seniors. Here's why it's pivotal:

1. Nutrient Variety: A balanced diet for seniors encompasses a wide array of nutrients, including vitamins, minerals, fiber, and antioxidants. This diversity of nutrients is crucial for maintaining overall health, bolstering the immune system, and promoting vitality.

2. Sustainable Weight Loss: The essence of balanced eating lies in creating a calorie deficit while ensuring that the body receives essential nutrients. This approach promotes gradual and sustainable weight loss, steering clear of crash diets that can be detrimental to health.

3. Sustaining Energy Levels: Seniors often require a consistent source of energy to fuel their daily activities and exercise routines. Balanced eating provides the necessary energy while maintaining a calorie deficit, which is essential for fat loss.

4. *Appetite Management:* A well-balanced diet with an adequate intake of proteins, carbohydrates, and fats can help control appetite and diminish cravings, which can be particularly helpful for seniors adhering to a weight loss plan.

5. *Digestive Health:* The inclusion of fiber-rich foods, such as whole grains, fruits, and vegetables, in a balanced diet supports healthy digestion. This can mitigate digestive issues and enhance comfort during weight-loss efforts.

The Role of Protein, Carbohydrates, and Fats

Understanding the functions of macronutrients is paramount for senior nutrition and effective weight management.

1. *Protein:* Seniors should prioritize adequate protein intake. Protein is the building block of muscle tissue and aids in muscle preservation, which is crucial during weight loss. Sources of lean protein, including lean meats, poultry, fish, dairy products, and plant-based options like beans and tofu, should be a part of their diet.

2. *Carbohydrates:* Carbohydrates are the body's primary energy source. Seniors should gravitate toward complex carbohydrates found in whole grains, fruits, vegetables, and legumes. These sources release energy gradually, providing a steady supply of energy throughout the day and assisting in maintaining stable blood sugar levels.

3. Fats: Healthy fats are indispensable for overall health. They play vital roles in brain function, hormone production, and the absorption of fat-soluble vitamins. Sources of healthy fats, such as avocados, nuts, seeds, and olive oil, should be incorporated into the diet in moderation.

Portion Control and Mindful Eating

Portion control and mindful eating are practical strategies for seniors embarking on a weight-loss journey.

1. Portion Control: Seniors should pay attention to portion sizes to prevent overconsumption of calories. Using smaller plates and utensils can visually guide appropriate portion sizes. Furthermore, reading food labels and understanding serving sizes can aid in portion control.

2. Mindful Eating: This practice encourages individuals to engage fully in the eating experience. Seniors should savor each bite, eat slowly, and cultivate an awareness of their body's hunger and fullness cues. By listening to their bodies, they can prevent overeating and make more conscious food choices.

3. *Emotional Eating Awareness:* Stress or other emotional triggers may cause emotional eating, which can impede weight loss. Seniors should strive to recognize these triggers and develop healthier coping mechanisms for managing emotional challenges without resorting to food.

4. *Hydration:* Adequate hydration is often underestimated, but it plays a crucial role in appetite regulation. Seniors should ensure they drink water regularly throughout the day to prevent thirst from being mistaken for hunger.

In summary, nutrition is a vital component of senior weight loss. A balanced diet rich in essential nutrients, an understanding of the roles of macronutrients, and the practice of portion control and mindful eating collectively lay a solid foundation for seniors to achieve and sustain a healthy weight.

CHAPTER 3

SENIOR-FRIENDLY WORKOUTS

Low-Impact Exercises for Seniors

Low-impact exercises are gentle on the joints and are highly beneficial for seniors due to their reduced risk of injury and suitability for various fitness levels. These exercises offer numerous advantages:

1. Joint Health: Low-impact exercises help maintain joint health by minimizing stress on the knees, hips, and spine. This is especially crucial for seniors, as joint-related issues become more common with age.

2. Improved Cardiovascular Health: Activities like walking, swimming, and cycling at a moderate pace can enhance cardiovascular fitness without placing excessive strain on the heart. This is vital for reducing the risk of heart disease.

3. Enhanced Balance and Coordination: Many low-impact exercises, such as tai chi and yoga, focus on balance and coordination. These activities can help seniors prevent falls and improve their overall stability.

4. Weight Management: Regular low-impact exercise can aid in weight management and fat loss by burning calories and increasing metabolism. This is particularly beneficial for seniors aiming to maintain a healthy weight.

5. *Stress Reduction:* Engaging in low-impact activities can reduce stress and improve mental well-being. Mindfulness-based exercises like tai chi and yoga also promote relaxation.

6. *Social Interaction:* Many low-impact exercises can be done in group settings, promoting social interaction and reducing feelings of isolation, which can be common among seniors.

7. *Flexibility and Range of Motion:* Exercises like stretching and yoga can enhance flexibility and maintain a full range of motion, making daily activities easier and reducing the risk of injury.

Strength Training for Fat Loss

Strength training, often associated with lifting weights or resistance exercises, is a valuable component of a senior's fitness routine, particularly for fat loss. Here's why:

1. *Increased Muscle Mass:* Strength training helps seniors build and maintain lean muscle mass. Muscle

tissue is metabolically active and burns more calories at rest, aiding in fat loss.

2. *Improved Metabolism:* As seniors age, their metabolism tends to slow down. Strength training can counteract this decline by increasing metabolism and helping to burn more calories throughout the day.

3. *Enhanced Mobility:* Strength training improves joint stability, bone density, and muscle strength, which in turn enhance mobility. This allows seniors to engage in more activities, promoting weight loss.

4. *Balanced Hormones:* Strength training can help regulate hormones, such as insulin, that play a role in fat storage. This can aid in weight loss and improve overall health.

5. *Fat Burning:* Strength training can lead to an afterburn effect, where the body continues to burn calories even after the workout is completed. This is especially beneficial for fat loss.

6. *Injury Prevention:* Building strength in key muscle groups can help prevent injuries that may otherwise hinder physical activity and weight loss efforts.

Cardiovascular Fitness for Seniors

Cardiovascular fitness, often referred to as cardio or aerobic exercise, is essential for seniors to maintain heart health and overall fitness. Here's why it's crucial:

1. Heart Health: Cardiovascular exercise strengthens the heart, improving its ability to pump blood efficiently. This reduces the risk of heart disease, a leading cause of mortality among seniors.

2. Improved Lung Function: Aerobic exercise enhances lung capacity, making it easier to breathe and increasing overall endurance.

3. Weight Management: Regular cardiovascular workouts help burn calories, aiding in weight management and fat loss when combined with a healthy diet.

4. Lowering Blood Pressure: Cardio exercises can lower blood pressure, reducing the risk of hypertension and its associated complications.

5. Enhanced Mood: Aerobic activities release endorphins, which can alleviate stress, anxiety, and depression—common concerns among seniors.

6. *Stamina and Energy:* Improved cardiovascular fitness leads to increased stamina and energy levels, allowing seniors to engage in daily activities with ease.

7. *Better Sleep:* Regular cardio workouts can improve sleep patterns, contributing to overall well-being.

CHAPTER 4

CREATING A PERSONALIZED SENIOR FAT LOSS PLAN

Assessing Your Current Health

Assessing your current health is a crucial first step in any fitness and nutrition journey. It provides a baseline understanding of your physical condition and helps you set realistic goals. Here's how to go about it:

1. Medical Check-Up: Begin by scheduling a comprehensive medical checkup with your healthcare provider. This should include measurements of vital signs like blood pressure, heart rate, and body mass index (BMI). It's also an opportunity to discuss any existing medical conditions, medications, or dietary restrictions.

2. Physical Fitness Assessment: Assess your current physical fitness level. This can include evaluating your flexibility, strength, endurance, and balance. You can perform basic exercises like the sit-and-reach test for flexibility or a simple walk to measure endurance.

3. Body Composition Analysis: Understanding your body composition is vital. This involves measuring your body fat percentage, which can be done using methods like skinfold calipers, bioelectrical impedance scales, or DEXA scans. This information helps tailor your fitness and nutrition plans.

4. Dietary Assessment: Keep a food diary for a few days to understand your eating habits. Note down everything you eat and drink, including portion sizes. This can provide insights into calorie intake, nutrient balance, and areas where dietary improvements are needed.

5. Goal Setting: Based on the gathered information and in consultation with your healthcare provider, set clear and realistic health and fitness goals. These goals should be specific, measurable, achievable, relevant, and time-bound (SMART).

Setting Calorie and Macronutrient Goals

Setting calorie and macronutrient goals is vital for achieving and maintaining a healthy weight. Here's how to do it:

1. Determine Total Daily Energy Expenditure (TDEE): Calculate your TDEE, which represents the total number of calories your body needs in a day to maintain its current weight. TDEE is influenced by factors like age, gender, weight, activity level, and metabolism.

2. Set a calorie deficit: To lose weight, create a calorie deficit by consuming fewer calories than your TDEE. A common guideline is to aim for a deficit of 500–1,000 calories per day, which can result in a safe and sustainable weight loss of about 1-2 pounds per week.

3. Establish Macronutrient Ratios: Determine the ideal macronutrient distribution for your diet. A balanced approach generally includes around 45–65% of calories from carbohydrates, 10–35% from protein, and 20–35% from healthy fats. Adjust these ratios based on your dietary preferences and goals.

4. Plan Meals: Design a meal plan that aligns with your calorie and macronutrient goals. Focus on nutrient-dense foods like fruits, vegetables, lean proteins, whole grains, and healthy fats. Ensure portion control to meet your calorie targets.

5. Track and monitor: Use tools like food diaries, apps, or online calculators to track your daily calorie and macronutrient intake. Regular monitoring helps you stay on track and make adjustments as needed.

Designing a Workout Routine

Designing an effective workout routine involves tailoring exercises to your fitness goals, physical condition, and preferences. Here's a step-by-step guide:

1. Set clear goals: Define your fitness objectives, whether it's weight loss, muscle gain, improved cardiovascular health, or enhanced flexibility. Your goals will guide your exercise choices.

2. Choose exercise types: Select a variety of exercises that align with your goals. For cardiovascular fitness, consider activities like walking, swimming, cycling, or dancing. For strength training, incorporate exercises for all major muscle groups.

3. Frequency and Duration: Determine how often you'll work out each week and the duration of each session. Gradually increase the intensity and duration as your fitness level improves.

4. Warm-Up and Cool-Down: Always begin with a warm-up to prepare your muscles and joints for exercise. End each session with a cool-down to gradually lower your heart rate and prevent injury.

5. *Progressive Overload:* To see improvements, gradually increase the intensity of your workouts. This can be achieved by lifting heavier weights, increasing repetitions, or extending the exercise duration.

6. *Rest and Recovery:* Allow your body adequate time to recover between workouts. Rest days are essential to prevent overtraining and promote muscle repair and growth.

7. *Flexibility and Balance:* Include flexibility and balance exercises, such as yoga or stretching routines, to maintain joint mobility and reduce the risk of injury.

8. *Stay consistent:* Consistency is key. Stick to your workout routine, but be flexible in adapting it to your changing needs and preferences over time.

CHAPTER 5

MEAL PLANNING FOR SENIORS

Building Healthy Meals

Day 1:

Breakfast:

- Greek yogurt with mixed berries and a drizzle of honey
- Whole-grain toast with almond butter

Lunch:

- Grilled chicken salad with mixed greens, cherry tomatoes, cucumbers, and balsamic vinaigrette dressing
- Quinoa or brown rice on the side

Dinner:

- Baked salmon with lemon and herbs
- Steamed broccoli
- Mashed sweet potatoes

Snack:

Sliced carrots and celery with hummus

Day 2:

Breakfast:

- Oatmeal topped with sliced banana, chopped nuts, and a sprinkle of cinnamon
- A boiled egg

Lunch:

- Lentil soup
- Whole-grain roll with a side of mixed greens and vinaigrette dressing

Dinner:

- Grilled shrimp skewers with a garlic and herb marinade
- Quinoa pilaf with sautéed spinach and cherry tomatoes

Snack:

- Greek yogurt with a handful of almonds

Day 3:

Breakfast:

- Whole-grain cereal with low-fat milk or a dairy-free alternative
- Fresh berries on top

Lunch:

- Turkey and avocado whole-grain wrap with spinach and mustard
- A side of sliced bell peppers

Dinner:

- Baked chicken breast with roasted asparagus and a squeeze of lemon
- Brown rice or cauliflower rice

Snack:

- Sliced apples with a tablespoon of peanut butter

Day 4:

Breakfast:

- Scrambled eggs with spinach, tomatoes, and feta cheese
- Whole-grain toast

Lunch:

- Mixed bean salad with bell peppers, red onion, and a lemon-tahini dressing
- Whole-grain crackers

Dinner:

- Baked cod with a dill and lemon sauce
- Quinoa or couscous
- Steamed green beans

Snack:

- A handful of mixed nuts

Day 5:

Breakfast:

- Smoothie with spinach, banana, Greek yogurt, and a scoop of protein powder

Lunch:

- Chickpea and vegetable stir-fry with a teriyaki sauce
- Brown rice

Dinner:

- Grilled tofu or chicken with a homemade pesto sauce
- Roasted Brussels sprouts

Snack:

- Cottage cheese with pineapple chunks

Day 6:

Breakfast:

- Whole-grain pancakes with fresh berries and a dollop of yogurt

Lunch:

- Spinach and quinoa salad with roasted beets, goat cheese, and balsamic glaze

Dinner:

- Beef or mushroom and vegetable kebabs with a Mediterranean-style couscous salad

Snack:

- Sliced cucumber with tzatziki sauce

Day 7:

Breakfast:

- Whole-grain waffles with sliced peaches and a drizzle of maple syrup
- A boiled egg

Lunch:

- Lentil and vegetable stew

- Whole-grain roll with a side of mixed greens and vinaigrette dressing

Dinner:

- Baked or grilled salmon with a citrus and herb marinade
- Quinoa with roasted broccoli and carrots

Snack:

- A small handful of grapes and a few cubes of cheese

Day 8:

Breakfast:

- Greek yogurt with mixed berries and a drizzle of honey
- Whole-grain toast with almond butter

Lunch:

- Grilled chicken salad with mixed greens, cherry tomatoes, cucumbers, and balsamic vinaigrette dressing
- Quinoa or brown rice on the side

Dinner:

- Baked salmon with lemon and herbs

- Steamed broccoli
- Mashed sweet potatoes

Snack:

Sliced carrots and celery with hummus

Day 9:

Breakfast:

- Oatmeal topped with sliced banana, chopped nuts, and a sprinkle of cinnamon
- A boiled egg

Lunch:

- Lentil soup
- Whole-grain roll with a side of mixed greens and vinaigrette dressing

Dinner:

- Grilled shrimp skewers with a garlic and herb marinade
- Quinoa pilaf with sautéed spinach and cherry tomatoes

Snack:

- Greek yogurt with a handful of almonds

Day 10:

Breakfast:

- Whole-grain cereal with low-fat milk or a dairy-free alternative
- Fresh berries on top

Lunch:

- Turkey and avocado whole-grain wrap with spinach and mustard
- A side of sliced bell peppers

Dinner:

- Baked chicken breast with roasted asparagus and a squeeze of lemon
- Brown rice or cauliflower rice

Snack:

- Sliced apples with a tablespoon of peanut butter

Day 11:

Breakfast:

- Scrambled eggs with spinach, tomatoes, and feta cheese
- Whole-grain toast

Lunch:

- Mixed bean salad with bell peppers, red onion, and a lemon-tahini dressing
- Whole-grain crackers

Dinner:

- Baked cod with a dill and lemon sauce
- Quinoa or couscous
- Steamed green beans

Snack: A handful of mixed nuts

Day 12:

Breakfast:

- Smoothie with spinach, banana, Greek yogurt, and a scoop of protein powder

Lunch:

- Chickpea and vegetable stir-fry with a teriyaki sauce
- Brown rice

Dinner:

- Grilled tofu or chicken with a homemade pesto sauce
- Roasted Brussels sprouts

40

Snack:

- Cottage cheese with pineapple chunks

Day 13:

Breakfast:

- Whole-grain pancakes with fresh berries and a dollop of yogurt

Lunch:

- Spinach and quinoa salad with roasted beets, goat cheese, and balsamic glaze

Dinner:

- Beef or mushroom and vegetable kebabs with a Mediterranean-style couscous salad

Snack: Sliced cucumber with tzatziki sauce

Day 14:

Breakfast:

- Whole-grain waffles with sliced peaches and a drizzle of maple syrup
- A boiled egg

Lunch:

- Lentil and vegetable stew

- Whole-grain roll with a side of mixed greens and vinaigrette dressing

Dinner:

- Baked or grilled salmon with a citrus and herb marinade
- Quinoa with roasted broccoli and carrots

Snack:

- A small handful of grapes and a few cubes of cheese

Meal Prep for Seniors

Meal prep is an excellent strategy for seniors to ensure they have convenient, nutritious, and balanced meals readily available. It can save time, promote healthier eating, and make it easier to maintain a consistent diet.

1. Plan Your Meals:

- Start by planning your meals for the week. Consider your dietary preferences, nutritional needs, and any dietary restrictions or health goals.
- Ensure a variety of foods, including lean proteins, whole grains, fruits, vegetables, and healthy fats.

2. Create a shopping list:

- Based on your meal plan, make a detailed shopping list to ensure you have all the necessary ingredients.

3. Choose Meal Prep Days:

- Select one or two days a week when you have time to dedicate to meal prep. Many people find Sunday and Wednesday to be convenient days for this.

4. Invest in containers:

- Purchase a variety of containers in different sizes, including airtight containers for storing prepared meals. Glass or BPA-free plastic containers are good options.

5. Prepare ingredients:

- Wash, peel, chop, and portion your ingredients. This can include vegetables, fruits, lean proteins, and grains.
- Cook grains like rice, quinoa, or pasta and let them cool before storing.

6. Cook proteins: Bake, grill, or poach proteins like chicken, fish, or tofu in bulk. Season them with herbs and spices for flavor.

- Divide cooked proteins into individual portions and store them in containers.

7. Cook vegetables:

- Roast or steam vegetables such as broccoli, carrots, and bell peppers. Season them lightly with olive oil, salt, and pepper.
- Portion vegetables into containers.

8. Prepare healthy snacks:

- Create healthy snack options, like cut-up fruit, yogurt, or a mix of nuts and dried fruits. Portion them into small containers or snack-sized bags.

9. Make sauces and dressings:

- Prepare sauces, dressings, or marinades that you can use throughout the week. Store them in small containers for easy access.

10. Assemble Meals:

- Based on your meal plan, assemble complete meals in containers. For example, combine a protein, a grain, and vegetables. Label containers with the date for reference.

11. Freeze Extra Portions:

- If you've prepared more food than you can consume within a few days, consider freezing individual portions for future use. Be sure to use freezer-safe containers.

12. Store Properly:

- Store your prepared meals and ingredients in the refrigerator or freezer, depending on how soon you plan to eat them.
- Properly label and date items for easy identification.

13. Reheat safely:

- When reheating meals, use a microwave or oven to ensure safe and even heating.
- Follow recommended guidelines for food safety, including reheating food to the appropriate temperature.

14. Stay Hydrated:

- Don't forget to include hydration in your meal prep plan. Fill water bottles or containers with water or herbal teas for easy access during the week.

15. Adapt and experiment:

- Be open to adapting your meal prep routine based on your evolving dietary needs, preferences, and feedback. Experiment with new recipes and ingredients to keep things interesting.

Special Dietary Considerations

"Special dietary considerations" refer to specific dietary needs or restrictions that individuals may have due to various factors, such as medical conditions, allergies, religious or cultural beliefs, ethical choices, or personal preferences. These considerations often require adjustments to one's regular diet to ensure it aligns with these unique requirements.

1. Medical Conditions:

- Many individuals have dietary needs driven by medical conditions. Common examples include:
- Diabetes: People with diabetes need to manage their carbohydrate intake to control blood sugar levels.
- Celiac Disease: Individuals with celiac disease must avoid gluten-containing foods to prevent intestinal damage.

- Hypertension: Those with high blood pressure often need to reduce their sodium (salt) intake to manage their condition.
- Food Allergies: Allergies to specific foods, such as peanuts or shellfish, require complete avoidance of those allergens.

2. Religious and Cultural Beliefs:

- Religious and cultural practices often dictate dietary restrictions and preferences. For instance:
- Halal: In Islam, adherents follow dietary laws that require specific preparation and avoidance of certain foods, like pork.
- Kosher: In Judaism, kosher dietary laws outline what foods are permissible and how they should be prepared.
- Vegetarianism: Some choose these diets for ethical or religious reasons, avoiding meat and animal products.

3. Ethical and Environmental Choices:

- Many people adopt special diets based on ethical concerns and environmental sustainability.
- Vegetarian: Avoids meat but may include other animal products like dairy and eggs.

- Veganism excludes all animal products, including dairy, eggs, and honey.
- Sustainable Diets: Focus on choosing foods with minimal environmental impact, such as reducing red meat consumption.

4. *Weight Management:*

- Special dietary considerations for weight management often involve monitoring calorie intake and nutrient balance. This includes diets for weight loss, weight gain, or maintaining a healthy weight.

5. *Age-Related Diets:*

- Infants, children, and the elderly often have specific dietary needs based on their developmental stage or age-related health concerns.
- Infants: exclusive breastfeeding or formula feeding with gradual introduction of solid foods
- Children: balanced diets for growth and development with age-appropriate portion sizes
- Seniors: Special considerations for maintaining bone health, managing chronic conditions, and ensuring proper nutrient intake

6. *Athletic and Performance Diets:*

- Athletes may follow special diets to optimize their performance, including diets high in carbohydrates for endurance or high in protein for muscle recovery.

7. *Specific Nutrient Requirements:*

- Certain conditions, such as iron-deficiency anemia or vitamin deficiencies, may require diets rich in specific nutrients.
- Iron Deficiency: Increased consumption of iron-rich foods like red meat, spinach, and beans
- Vitamin D Deficiency: Foods rich in vitamin D, like fortified dairy products and fatty fish,

8. *Allergen Avoidance:*

- Some individuals have allergies to common foods, requiring strict avoidance of the allergen(s).
- Peanut Allergy: Total avoidance of peanuts and peanut products
- Gluten Allergy: Complete Avoidance of Gluten-Containing Foods

9. Medical Procedures and Treatments:

- Certain medical procedures or treatments may necessitate specific dietary restrictions or modifications.
- Post-Surgery: After certain surgeries, such as bariatric surgery, a liquid or soft diet may initially be required.
- Chemotherapy: Patients may experience changes in taste and appetite, requiring modifications to their diet.

10. Gastrointestinal Conditions:

- Conditions like irritable bowel syndrome (IBS) or inflammatory bowel disease (IBD) may require diets that reduce trigger foods to manage symptoms.

CHAPTER 6

STAYING MOTIVATED AND OVERCOMING OBSTACLES

Setting realistic expectations

1. Understand Your Starting Point: Knowing where you currently stand in terms of your fitness, weight, and overall health is the first step. This baseline assessment allows you to set goals that are achievable and relevant to your personal situation.

2. Set SMART Goals: SMART goals are specific, measurable, achievable, relevant, and time-bound. Here's a breakdown:

- *Specific:* Clearly define your goal. Instead of saying, "I want to lose weight," specify, "I want to lose 10 pounds."
- *Measurable:* Make sure you can track your progress. Use metrics like weight, body measurements, or fitness performance.
- *Achievable:* Your goal should be realistic within your circumstances. Losing 10 pounds in a month may not be achievable or healthy, but over three to four months is more realistic.

- *Relevant:* Your goal should align with your broader objectives, such as improving overall health or enhancing fitness.
- *Time-bound:* Set a timeframe for achieving your goal, which adds urgency and motivation.

3. Prioritize health and wellness: Shift your mindset away from solely focusing on the number on the scale. Place importance on health improvements such as increased energy levels, better sleep, reduced stress, and enhanced mood. These small victories can provide significant motivation.

4. Research Realistic Rates: Understanding what constitutes healthy and sustainable progress is crucial. Rapid weight loss diets or extreme workout routines are often unsustainable and can be detrimental to your health. Aim for a gradual weight loss of 1-2 pounds per week, which is generally considered safe and sustainable.

5. Celebrate non-scale victories: While the scale is one measure of progress, it doesn't capture all your achievements. Celebrate milestones like improved stamina, flexibility, or endurance in your workouts.

Recognize healthier food choices and the development of sustainable habits.

6. *Be Patient:* Transforming your body and health is a long-term endeavor. Resist the urge to resort to quick-fix solutions, which often lead to short-lived results and potential health risks. Understand that sustainable change takes time and commitment.

7. *Adapt and Adjust:* As you progress, your goals may evolve. You might find that your initial goal of losing weight transitions into maintaining your current weight while increasing muscle mass. Be open to adjusting your expectations based on what you learn about your body and what makes you feel your best.

Dealing with Plateaus

1. *Stay calm and patient.* Plateaus are a natural part of any fitness journey. They can be discouraging, but it's essential to remain patient and maintain a positive attitude. Remember that plateaus are temporary.

2. *Evaluate Your Routine:* When you hit a plateau, it's a good time to assess your current workout and nutrition plan. Ask yourself if you're still challenging yourself during workouts and if your eating habits could be more balanced.

3. *Change up your workouts:* Introducing variety into your exercise routine can help break through plateaus. Try different exercises, increase the intensity or duration of your workouts, or consider incorporating new forms of physical activity.

4. *Adjust nutrition:* Reevaluating your calorie and macronutrient intake can be beneficial. Small adjustments, such as modifying portion sizes or experimenting with nutrient timing, can sometimes jumpstart progress.

5. *Monitor Progress:* It's crucial to track more than just your weight. Measure your body, pay attention to how your clothes fit, and record your fitness achievements. These metrics can reveal progress that the scale might not show.

6. *Rest and Recovery:* Overtraining can contribute to plateaus. Ensure you're giving your body enough time to recover between workouts. This includes both physical and mental recovery.

7. *Set mini-goals:* Breaking down your larger fitness or weight loss goals into smaller, achievable milestones can provide motivation and a sense of progress. Celebrate these mini-goals as you achieve them.

8. *Stay Consistent:* It's easy to become disheartened and consider giving up during plateaus, but consistency is key to overcoming them. Continue to adhere to your routine and make adjustments as needed. Consistency often leads to breakthroughs.

Staying Consistent:

1. *Establish a Routine:* Create a structured schedule for your workouts, meals, and sleep. Consistency in your daily habits can lead to long-term success.

2. *Find enjoyment:* Choose physical activities and exercises that you genuinely enjoy. When you look forward to your workouts, you're more likely to stick with them over the long term.

3. *Set Reminders:* Life can get busy, and it's easy to forget your fitness and nutrition commitments. Use reminders, alarms, or calendar notifications to prompt you to exercise or prepare healthy meals.

4. *Create accountability:* Partner up with a friend, family member, or workout buddy. Joining fitness classes, groups, or online communities can provide accountability and social support, helping you stay motivated.

5. *Track Progress:* Keeping a record of your workouts, meals, and achievements can help you see your progress over time. It can be motivating to look back and realize how far you've come.

6. *Practice self-compassion*. Recognize that perfection is not required for progress. If you miss a workout or indulge in a treat occasionally, don't be too hard on yourself. Focus on long-term consistency rather than momentary lapses.

7. *Visualize Success:* Spend time visualizing how you'll feel and look when you achieve your fitness and weight loss goals. Visualization can boost motivation and determination.

8. *Adapt to Life Changes:* Life is dynamic, and unexpected events can disrupt your routine. When this happens, adapt and get back on track as soon as possible. Flexibility is key to maintaining consistency.

9. *Reward Yourself:* Celebrate your achievements, whether they're big or small. Rewards can help reinforce your commitment and provide positive reinforcement for your efforts.

10. Remember Your "Why: Reflect on the reasons you started your fitness and weight loss journey. Keeping your motivations in mind can help you stay committed, especially during challenging times.

In summary, setting realistic expectations, effectively managing plateaus, and maintaining consistency are integral to achieving your fitness and weight loss goals. Approaching your journey with patience, adaptability, and a focus on long-term health and well-being will increase your chances of success and make your efforts more enjoyable and sustainable.

CHAPTER 7

TRACKING PROGRESS

The importance of measurement cannot be overstated, as it plays a crucial role in various aspects of our lives, from science and engineering to everyday tasks. Here are several key reasons why measurement is essential:

1. Accurate Data and Information: Measurement provides a standardized way to gather accurate data and information. Whether in scientific research, healthcare, or manufacturing, precise measurements help ensure that data is reliable and trustworthy. This accuracy forms the foundation for informed decision-making.

2. Quality Control: In manufacturing and production, precise measurements are vital for maintaining quality control. By measuring the dimensions, tolerances, and properties of products, manufacturers can ensure consistency and meet quality standards. This is critical for the safety and functionality of products.

3. Safety: Measurements are essential for safety in various contexts. For example, accurate measurements of medication doses are crucial to preventing medical errors. In construction and engineering, precise measurements ensure the structural integrity and safety of buildings and infrastructure.

4. *Scientific Discovery:* Science relies heavily on measurement. It enables scientists to quantify and analyze natural phenomena, leading to discoveries and a deeper understanding of the natural world. Measurements underpin scientific theories, experiments, and research.

5. *Engineering and Design:* Engineers use measurements extensively in the design and construction of structures, machinery, electronics, and more. Accurate measurements are essential for ensuring that designs are functional, safe, and efficient.

6. *Healthcare and Medicine:* In healthcare, measurements of vital signs, lab values, and medical imaging play a critical role in diagnosing illnesses, monitoring patient health, and guiding treatment decisions. Precise measurements are essential for patient safety and care.

7. *Environmental Monitoring:* Measurement is crucial for assessing and monitoring environmental conditions such as air quality, water quality, and climate data.

Accurate measurements inform environmental policies, conservation efforts, and disaster preparedness.

8. *Financial Transactions:* Measurements of currency, time, and quantities are fundamental to financial transactions and economic activities. Accurate measurements are essential for fair trade and commerce.

9. *Education:* Measurements are a fundamental part of education, helping students understand and apply concepts related to length, weight, time, and more. They are also used in educational assessments to evaluate student performance.

10. *Progress Tracking:* In personal and professional development, measurements help individuals track progress and set goals. Whether it's monitoring fitness, tracking financial goals, or assessing academic performance, measurements provide tangible benchmarks for improvement.

11. *Communication and Standardization:* Measurements provide a common language for communication. Standard units of measurement, such as the metric system, ensure consistency and facilitate communication across different regions and industries.

12. *Problem Solving:* Measurements are essential for solving practical problems. Whether it's determining the right amount of ingredients for a recipe, measuring distances for travel, or assessing the energy consumption of appliances, measurements help us find solutions.

13. *Innovation:* Measurement advancements often lead to innovation. New measurement technologies and tools enable the development of more efficient processes, improved products, and novel solutions to existing challenges.

Using Technology for Monitoring

Technology has revolutionized the way we monitor progress, making it more accessible and efficient. Here's how to harness the power of technology for effective monitoring:

1. *Select the Right Tools:* Begin by choosing the technology tools and apps that align with your specific goals. There are a wide range of options available, including fitness trackers, health apps, goal-setting apps, and more. For instance, if you're monitoring fitness, a fitness tracker like a smartwatch can be invaluable.

2. Set clear metrics: define the key metrics you want to monitor. These could be related to health, fitness, financial goals, or any area of personal development. For health, this might include steps taken, calorie intake, or sleep patterns.

3. Input Accurate Data: Ensure that you input accurate data into your chosen technology tools. For example, if you're tracking your expenses with a budgeting app, diligently enter all your income and expenditures to get an accurate financial picture.

4. Regularly update data: consistency is key to effective monitoring. Make it a habit to update your data regularly. This could mean syncing your fitness tracker daily, recording your meals, or inputting your savings and expenses.

5. Set Reminders: Use reminders and notifications to prompt you to update or check your progress. Many apps allow you to set reminders for specific tasks or goals, helping you stay on track.

6. Analyze Trends: Most technology tools provide features for analyzing your data over time. Use these features to identify trends, patterns, and areas where you're making progress or need to adjust your efforts.

7. *Adjust Goals:* Based on the insights you gain from your technology tools, be willing to adjust your goals or strategies as needed. For instance, if your fitness tracker reveals that you're consistently falling short of your daily step goal, you might increase your daily activity.

8. *Seek Insights and Feedback:* Many apps and tools offer insights and feedback on your progress. Pay attention to these insights, as they can provide valuable guidance on areas for improvement.

9. *Sync Multiple Devices:* If you use multiple devices or apps for monitoring, ensure they can sync data with each other. This integration can provide a more comprehensive view of your progress.

Celebrating Achievements

Celebrating achievements is a crucial part of maintaining motivation and a positive mindset on your journey toward your goals. Here's how to celebrate your accomplishments effectively:

1. *Definition of Milestones:* Break your long-term goals into smaller, more achievable milestones. These could be weekly, monthly, or even daily accomplishments. For instance, if your goal is to lose 20 pounds, celebrate every 5-pound milestone.

2. *Choose Meaningful Rewards:* Select rewards that resonate with you and are meaningful. These could be treats like a favorite dessert, leisure activities like a movie night, or non-material rewards like time spent doing a hobby you love.

3. *Plan in Advance:* Plan your rewards in advance. Knowing what you'll treat yourself to when you achieve a milestone can be motivating in itself.

4. *Share Achievements:* Share your accomplishments with a supportive friend, family member, or online community. Celebrating with others can amplify the joy and sense of achievement.

5. *Document Achievements:* Keep a record of your achievements, whether it's through journaling, photos, or notes on your phone. Looking back at your successes can boost your confidence and motivation.

6. *Reflect on Progress:* Take time to reflect on how far you've come. Acknowledge the effort and dedication you've put into reaching your goals.

7. *Set New Goals:* After celebrating an achievement, set new goals or adjust existing ones. This ensures that you continue to challenge yourself and maintain your motivation.

8. *Maintain Balance:* While it's important to celebrate achievements, avoid overindulging in rewards that may hinder your progress. Balance celebration with a commitment to your ongoing journey.

CHAPTER 8

MAINTAINING WEIGHT LOSS AND A HEALTHY LIFESTYLE

Transitioning to Maintenance

1. Gradual Caloric Adjustments: Transitioning to maintenance requires you to find your new equilibrium for calorie intake. It's essential to make these adjustments slowly and mindfully. Sudden increases in calorie consumption can lead to unwanted weight regain.

2. Monitor Portion Sizes: While you're no longer focused on losing weight, portion control remains vital. Continue to be aware of portion sizes to avoid overeating. You can use tools like measuring cups and food scales to help with this.

3. Maintain a Balanced Diet: Continue to prioritize a balanced diet rich in fruits, vegetables, lean proteins, whole grains, and healthy fats. Be cautious of falling into the trap of thinking you can now eat anything you want. A balanced diet is not just for weight loss; it's essential for long-term health.

4. Regular Physical Activity: Transitioning to maintenance doesn't mean you can stop exercising.

Regular physical activity is crucial for maintaining not only your weight but also your overall health. Consider setting new fitness goals, such as improving your cardiovascular fitness, lifting heavier weights, or learning a new sport.

5. *Mindful Eating:* Mindful eating remains an essential practice during maintenance. Continue to listen to your body's hunger and fullness cues. It's easy to overindulge or eat out of habit, so stay present during meals and snacks.

6. *Regular Monitoring:* Don't abandon regular monitoring. While you don't need to track your calorie intake as meticulously as during weight loss, it's still valuable to occasionally check in on your progress. If you notice small weight fluctuations, it's a signal to reevaluate your eating and exercise habits.

7. *Set realistic expectations:* Understand that your weight may naturally fluctuate slightly, even during maintenance. This is entirely normal and doesn't indicate a failure. Embrace these fluctuations as part of your journey to long-term health.

8. *Celebrate Success:* Transitioning to maintenance is an achievement in itself. Celebrate this transition and use it as an opportunity to reflect on how far you've come in your health and fitness journey.

preventing weight gain

1. Stay Active: Physical activity remains your ally in preventing weight gain. The more muscle mass you maintain, the higher your resting metabolic rate, which makes it easier to control your weight. Make exercise a lifelong commitment.

2. Mindful Eating: Continue practicing mindful eating to prevent overeating and emotional eating. Pay attention to your body's hunger and fullness signals and use them as guides for your eating habits.

3. Set realistic goals: If you have further weight loss goals, approach them with patience and realistic expectations. Avoid drastic diets or exercise plans that promise rapid results. Slow, sustainable progress is the key.

4. Regular Monitoring: Even if you've reached your goal weight, monitoring your weight and health indicators can help you catch any deviations early. Early intervention is often more effective in preventing significant weight regain.

5. *Build a Support System:* Your support system remains crucial. Friends, family, or a weight loss group can provide encouragement and help you stay accountable.

6. *Healthy Environment:* Maintain an environment that supports your healthy lifestyle. Continue to keep your kitchen stocked with nutritious foods and minimize the availability of high-calorie, low-nutrient snacks.

7. *Stress Management:* Stress can lead to emotional eating and weight gain. Prioritize stress management techniques that work for you, whether it's meditation, yoga, or simply spending time in nature.

8. *Regular Sleep:* Ensure you get enough sleep consistently. Poor sleep patterns can disrupt your metabolism and lead to weight gain. Prioritize sleep as part of your long-term health strategy.

Long-Term Health and Wellness

1. *Regular health checkups:* Schedule regular checkups with your healthcare provider, even when you're feeling healthy. These appointments are essential for the early detection and prevention of health issues.

2. *Nutrient-Rich Diet:* Continue to educate yourself about nutrition and maintain a diet that provides essential nutrients. As you age, your nutrient needs may change, so it's important to adapt your diet accordingly.

3. *Physical Activity:* View physical activity as a lifelong commitment to health and well-being. Explore various forms of exercise to keep things interesting and maintain your fitness levels.

4. *Stress Reduction:* Managing stress isn't just essential for weight maintenance; it's crucial for overall health. Chronic stress can contribute to various health problems, including heart disease, anxiety, and depression.

5. *Social Connections:* Maintain and nurture your social connections. Loneliness and social isolation can have adverse effects on mental and physical health.

6. *Hydration:* Drinking an adequate amount of water daily remains essential. Proper hydration supports digestion, circulation, temperature regulation, and numerous other bodily functions.

7. *Rest and Recovery:* Prioritize rest and recovery as part of your overall health strategy. This includes not only sleep but also relaxation and leisure activities that rejuvenate you.

8. *Mindfulness and Self-Care:* Continue to practice mindfulness and self-care. Self-compassion and self-reflection are powerful tools for maintaining mental and emotional well-being.

9. *Continuous Learning:* Stay curious and open to new information and developments in health and wellness. Science and research are continually evolving, and staying informed empowers you to make informed choices.

CHAPTER 9

SENIOR-SPECIFIC CHALLENGES AND SOLUTIONS

Dealing with arthritis and joint pain

Arthritis and joint pain can be common challenges as we age. Here are strategies to help you manage and cope with these issues:

1. Pain Management: Work with your healthcare provider to develop a pain management plan. This may include medication, physical therapy, or lifestyle modifications.

2. Maintain a healthy weight: Excess weight can exacerbate joint pain, especially in weight-bearing joints like the knees and hips. Achieving and maintaining a healthy weight can help reduce the stress on your joints.

3. Exercise regularly: Engage in low-impact exercises that are easy on the joints, such as swimming, cycling, or tai chi. These activities can help maintain joint flexibility and reduce pain.

4. Joint-Friendly Diet: Consume an anti-inflammatory diet rich in fruits, vegetables, whole grains, and healthy fats. Omega-3 fatty acids found in fatty fish, flaxseeds, and walnuts may help reduce inflammation.

5. *Physical Therapy:* Consider physical therapy to improve joint function and reduce pain. A physical therapist can provide exercises and techniques tailored to your specific needs.

6. *Heat and cold therapy:* applying heat or cold packs to the affected joints can provide relief. Heat can relax muscles and increase blood flow, while cold can reduce inflammation and numb pain.

7. *Assistive Devices:* Depending on the severity of your joint issues, assistive devices like braces, splints, or canes may help reduce pain and improve mobility.

8. *Medications:* If prescribed, take medications as directed by your healthcare provider. These may include pain relievers, anti-inflammatories, or disease-modifying drugs for certain types of arthritis.

9. *Manage stress:* Stress can exacerbate pain. Practice stress-reduction techniques such as deep breathing, meditation, or mindfulness to help manage both physical and emotional discomfort.

Coping with Age-Related Stressors

As we age, various stressors can arise. Here are strategies to cope effectively with age-related stressors:

1. Maintain a Support System: Stay connected with friends and family. Social support is crucial for coping with stressors, as it provides a sense of belonging and emotional assistance.

2. Stay Active: Regular physical activity can help reduce stress and improve mood. Exercise releases endorphins, which are natural stress-relievers.

3. Practice relaxation techniques: Incorporate relaxation techniques into your daily routine, such as deep breathing exercises, progressive muscle relaxation, or yoga.

4. Maintain a Healthy Lifestyle: Prioritize a balanced diet, adequate sleep, and regular health checkups. These factors contribute to overall well-being and resilience to stress.

5. Set realistic expectations: Be kind to yourself and set realistic expectations. Understand that aging comes with changes, and it's okay to adapt and adjust your goals and activities.

6. Engage in Hobbies: Pursue hobbies and interests that bring you joy and fulfillment. Engaging in activities you're passionate about can be a great stress reliever.

7. Time Management: Organize your time effectively to reduce feelings of overwhelm. Prioritize tasks, delegate when possible, and make time for self-care.

8. Mindfulness and Meditation: Practice mindfulness and meditation to stay present and reduce rumination about past or future stressors.

9. Positive Thinking: Foster a positive outlook by focusing on gratitude and positive affirmations. Optimism can help you navigate challenges with resilience.

Medicine and Its Impact on Weight

Medications can sometimes have an impact on weight. Here's how to manage this aspect of your health:

1. Understand Side Effects: Learn about the potential side effects of your medications. Some drugs may affect appetite, metabolism, or water retention, which can lead to weight changes.

2. Balanced Diet: Focus on a balanced diet even while taking medication. Pay attention to portion sizes and make healthy food choices to manage your weight effectively.

3. *Stay Active:* Regular physical activity can help offset medication-related weight gain. It can also improve mood and overall well-being.

4. *Monitor Weight:* Keep track of your weight and any changes that occur after starting or adjusting medication. This information can be valuable for discussions with your healthcare provider.

5. *Medication Management:* Take your medications as prescribed by your healthcare provider. Never alter your dosage or stop taking a medication without their guidance.

6. *Explore Medication Alternatives:* If weight gain is a significant concern, discuss with your healthcare provider whether there are alternative medications with fewer side effects.

7. *Lifestyle Modifications:* Consider making lifestyle modifications to counteract medication-related weight gain. This might include dietary adjustments or additional exercise.

8. *Patient Advocacy:* Be an advocate for your own health. If you believe a medication is causing unwanted weight changes, don't hesitate to discuss your concerns with your healthcare provider and explore potential solutions.

CONCLUSION

It's clear that you're on a remarkable journey towards better health and well-being. You've explored essential topics like setting realistic goals, using technology for monitoring, and dealing with specific challenges such as arthritis and age-related stressors. Your dedication to lifelong learning and self-improvement is truly commendable.

As you continue along your path, remember that your health is a precious asset, and your well-being is worth every effort you invest. Embrace each day as an opportunity for growth, and face challenges with resilience and determination.

In your pursuit of a healthier and more fulfilling life, you've gained valuable insights into maintaining weight, managing stress, and optimizing your overall health. These insights will serve as valuable tools as you navigate the complexities of modern life.

Always prioritize self-care and self-compassion. Your journey may have its ups and downs, but it's your commitment to your well-being that truly matters. Celebrate every achievement, no matter how small, and remember that every step forward is a victory.

Your willingness to seek knowledge and take action to improve your life is an inspiration. Keep asking questions, keep exploring, and keep growing. Your future is filled with potential, and with each passing day, you're crafting a healthier, happier, and more vibrant you.

Here's to your continued success on this incredible journey towards better health and well-being. Your commitment to self-improvement is something to be proud of, and I have every confidence that your future will be filled with wellness, vitality, and fulfillment.

Manufactured by Amazon.ca
Acheson, AB